Introduction

This is the fourth in the **MyBones** series of co physicians authored by board-certified orth focuses on a specific area: neck, back, hip, knee, shoulder, elbow, hand, ankle, and foot along with several other topics that could be helpful to you. Please search on Amazon.com from time to time to see if a **MyBones** book addressing your area of concern has become available.

Medical science is complicated. When doctors talk, we use language foreign to most people, even those highly educated in other disciplines. Intelligent people want to understand their medical problems. We intend for this booklet to provide you and your loved ones a better understanding of your diagnosis and treatment options.

Two seasoned orthopaedic surgeons combine over 100 years of training and experience to help demystify the language of their profession. Moreover, they offer opinions about how they would wish their loved ones and themselves to be treated.

We believe this information will help you better communicate with your physician and will enable you to ask relevant questions to get useful answers. We want you to avoid problems when possible and take an active role in helping your surgeon determine the best course to follow when help is needed.

Our training after university consisted of four years of medical school followed by five years of specialized training in orthopaedic surgery under intense supervision. After two years in the United States Navy, one went into academic surgery where he practiced orthopaedic surgery and trained future surgeons. After two years as an orthopaedic surgeon in the United States Air Force, the other joined a group of orthopaedic surgeons in private practice.

We take full responsibility for what we say, but you need to understand that we are expressing our opinions based on training and experience. Medical science changes rapidly, so what seems to be true today may not be so tomorrow. Furthermore, it is common for medical people to have different opinions, so your surgeon's opinion may not be the same as ours. We are telling you what we think and believe to be true.

Reading this booklet does not make one an expert in the field. It cannot take the place of professional, in-person consultation. If your condition is persistent or worsening or you need more specific information about your case, please see an orthopaedic surgeon as soon as possible.

Be enlightened! Be empowered! Be healthy!

Table of Contents and Overview

Chapter 1: Spine Anatomy

In order to understand the diseases and disorders that occur in the neck, a review of spine anatomy and commonly used terms is provided.

Chapter 2: Commonly Used Imaging and Other Tests

Several imaging studies and tests are used to evaluate spine disorders and diseases.

Chapter 3: Non-Surgical Options of Neck Care

Various medications, injections, physical therapy, bracing, and pain management are discussed.

Chapter 4: Common Disorders Affecting the Neck

"Pinched nerves", *cervical radiculopathy,* may be caused by a herniated disc and/or degenerative disc disease. Compression of the spinal cord, *cervical myelopathy* due to *cervical spinal stenosis,* results in loss of balance, dexterity, and motor function.

Chapter 5: Arthritis, Cancer of the Spine, Spine Infections, and Spine Fractures

Rheumatoid arthritis and ankylosing spondylitis involving the neck are very disabling. Lung, breast and prostate cancer may spread to the cervical spine. Other types of tumors may originate in the spine and the spinal nerves. In order to treat infections, antibiotics coupled with surgical treatment are often needed. Neck fractures may require surgery.

Chapter 6: Complications of Neck Surgery

Surgical complications and the measures taken to avoid them are discussed.

Chapter 7: What to Expect after Your Surgery

 During the last decade, spine surgery has evolved to provide better outcomes through improved diagnostic techniques, less invasive procedures and use of modern implants.

Glossary

Medical terms and phrases are defined to help you better understand the conditions and treatments discussed.

Acknowledgements

We appreciate those who have inspired and helped us in this undertaking.

About the Authors

Reviewer Comments

Chapter 1: Spine Anatomy

In order to understand the abnormalities that can occur in your spine, it is helpful to first understand normal spine anatomy and terminology.

The spinal column is made up of thirty-three (33) vertebrae joined together by very strong ligaments and the intervertebral discs. There are seven (7) cervical, twelve (12) thoracic and five (5) lumbar vertebrae. The five (5) sacral vertebrae form a single block of bone, not separated by intervertebral discs as are the other vertebrae. The coccygeal vertebrae are small and considered remnants of a tail.

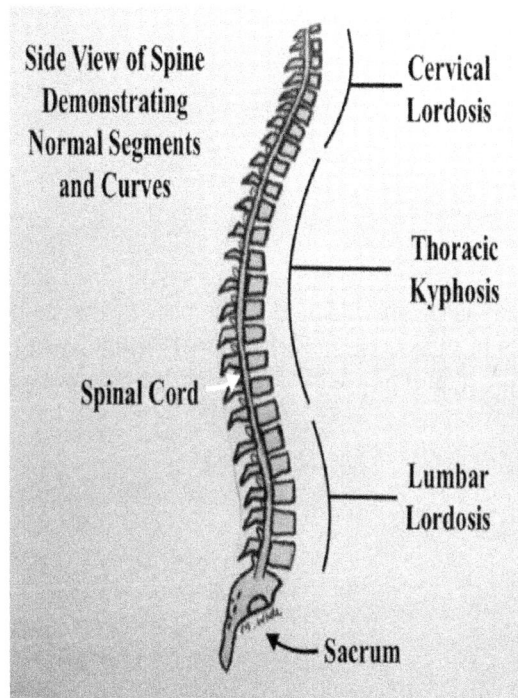

Side View of Spine Demonstrating Normal Segments and Curves

Cervical Lordosis

Thoracic Kyphosis

Spinal Cord

Lumbar Lordosis

Sacrum

When you are standing, you will notice that your cervical spine has a gentle forward curve, which positions your head over your shoulders. This is referred to as a *lordotic* curve. The thoracic spine has a backward curve, which is referred to as a *kyphotic* curve. The lumbar spine, like the cervical, has a lordotic curve. A spine lacking these normal curves is unable to provide normal posture and balance.

Ligaments of the Cervical Spine

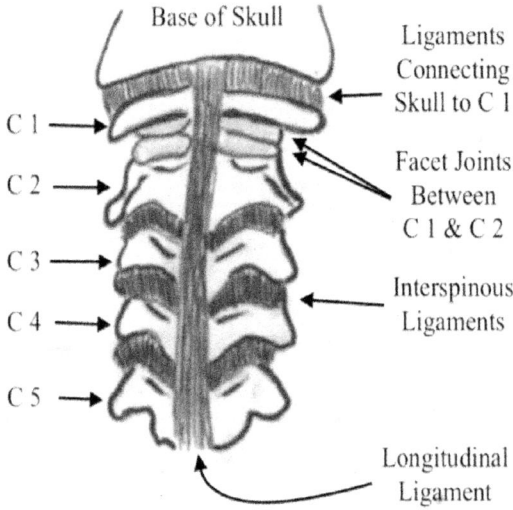

Base of Skull

Ligaments
Connecting
Skull to C 1

Facet Joints
Between
C 1 & C 2

Interspinous
Ligaments

Longitudinal
Ligament

C 1

C 2

C 3

C 4

C 5

The seven vertebrae of the cervical spine are attached to the base of the skull with very firm and strong ligaments. Even so, it is the most flexible part of the spine, making it the most vulnerable to injury.

Unique Relationship of C1 to C2

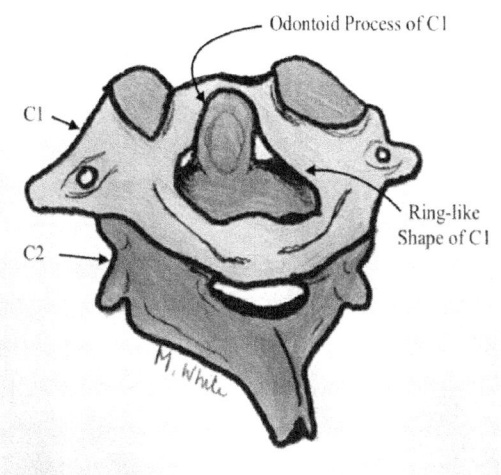

The upper two cervical vertebrae are unique in that the first cervical vertebra provides a ring-like shape to accommodate a peg, the *odontoid process*, projecting upward from the second cervical vertebra. This allows one to rotate the neck in a circular motion.

Each vertebra is made up of a cylinder of bone, *vertebral body*, arches, *pedicles*, and roof-like coverings, *laminae*, with an attached *spinous process*. These bony structures support, encase and protect the spinal cord and its nerves in the *spinal canal*.

Anatomy of a
Cervical Vertebra

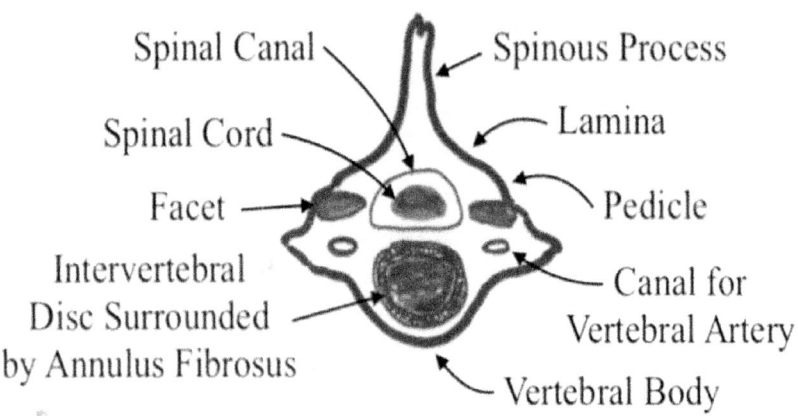

The spinal nerves exit the *spinal canal* through a window called a *foramen* located between vertebrae above and below it. Upper and lower projections called *facets* and the small joints of Luscha on the sides of the vertebrae provide attachment points between vertebrae. Each intervertebral disc is composed of a soft gelatinous interior, *the nucleus,* supported by strong interlacing ligaments, the *annulus fibrosus* that provide firm interconnections to the vertebral bodies.

Nerve Roots Exiting the Spine
Frontal View

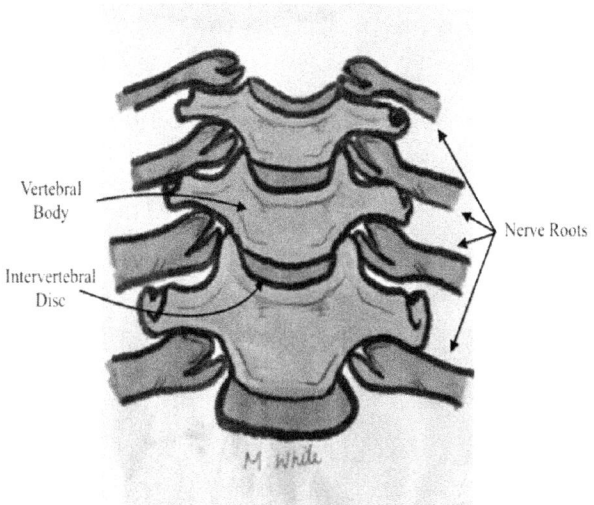

Vertebral
Body

Nerve Roots

Intervertebral
Disc

M. While

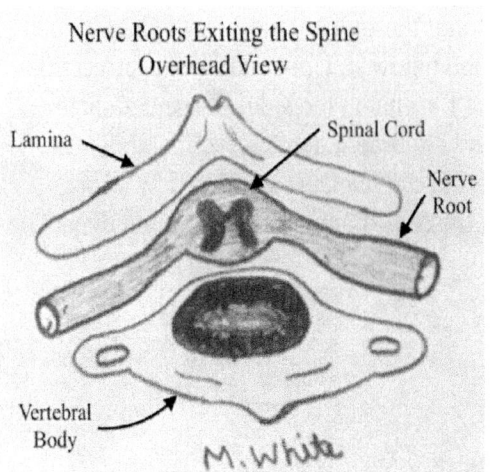

Nerve Roots Exiting the Spine
Overhead View

Lamina

Spinal Cord

Nerve
Root

Vertebral
Body

M.White

In order to relieve pressure on the spinal cord or nerve roots, it is usually necessary to remove a portion of the lamina to obtain access to the spinal cord and nerve roots. This can be a full laminectomy or a partial laminectomy, *hemilaminectomy*, in which only one side of the lamina is removed.

Cervical Laminectomy
Exposing the Dura Mater

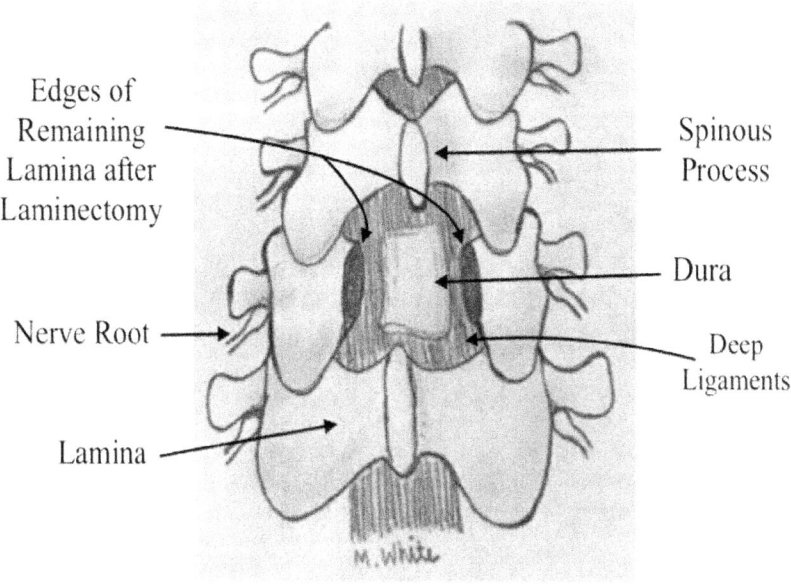

Edges of Remaining Lamina after Laminectomy

Spinous Process

Dura

Nerve Root

Deep Ligaments

Lamina

M. White

Posterior View

Partial Laminectomy
Posterior View

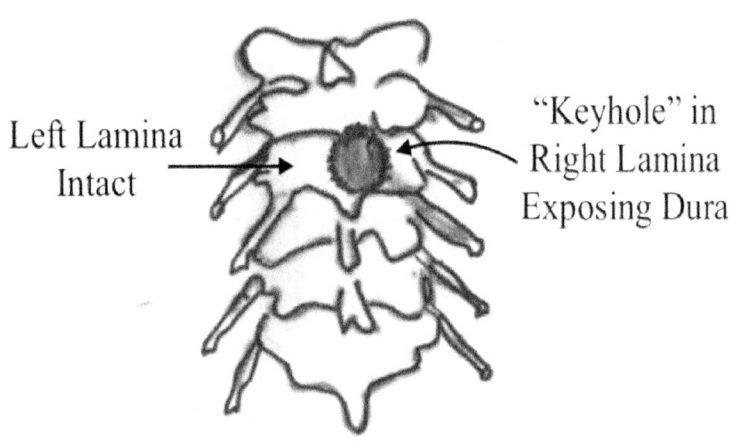

Left Lamina Intact

"Keyhole" in Right Lamina Exposing Dura

Partial Cervical Laminectomy
to Remove Herniated Disc
Overhead View

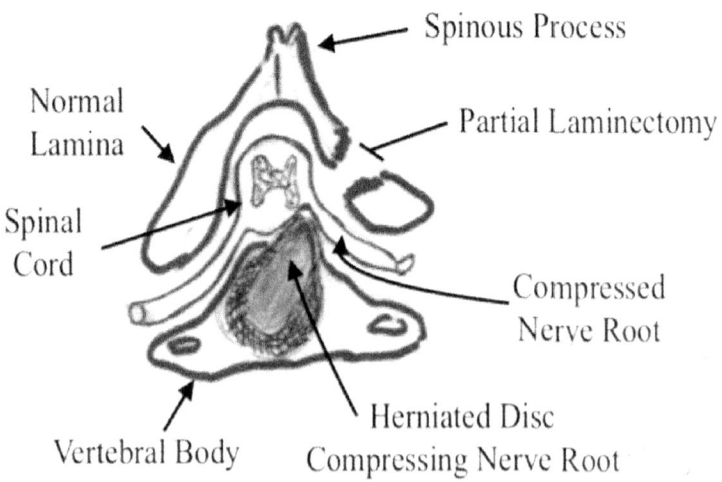

Spinous Process

Normal Lamina

Partial Laminectomy

Spinal Cord

Compressed Nerve Root

Vertebral Body

Herniated Disc Compressing Nerve Root

Chapter 2: Commonly Used Imaging and Other Studies

Spine surgeons rely on several types of imaging studies to guide them when making a diagnosis and planning treatment. Commonly performed X-Rays of the spine include front, side and oblique views. Bending films are useful in determining abnormal movements of vertebrae, unstable areas and flexibility of the spine.

Bone scans are performed by injecting a small amount of radioactive material into the patient. A scan of the skeleton is then done to detect areas of abnormal accumulation of the radioactive material, which occurs in patients with infections, tumors and fractures.

In order to evaluate your bone density measurement, a DEXA, dual energy x-ray absorption scan, using low dose X-ray beams is done. A **T score** shows the amount of bone you have compared with a young adult of the same gender with optimal bone mass. A T score above -1 is considered normal. A T-score between -1 and -2.5 is classified as **osteopenia**, often called "thin bones"). A T-score below -2.5 is defined as **osteoporosis**, often called "soft bones" or fragile bones, which is a high risk for fractures from minimal trauma.

Computerized tomography, **CT scan**, are computer modulated x-rays that allow visualization of the spine in three dimensions. CT scans can be done rapidly and are most helpful in evaluating patients with spinal fractures and tumors. They are often done after the introduction of dye into the fluid surrounding the spinal cord and nerves, *myelogram*, to visualize these structures.

In contrast to CT scans, Magnetic Radiographic Imaging, **MRI,** uses high strength electromagnets rather than radiation to image the spine. These studies provide useful information in making a diagnosis and planning treatment. The MRI provides visualization of bone and soft tissues such as ligaments, discs, and neural structures from the front, side and along the cross-sectional planes of the spine that cannot be visualized in any other way. CT and MRI are used in surgery to guide the surgeon and to verify placement of implants and instrumentation.

Electromyography, **EMG**, detects abnormal nerve and muscle function by sampling the response of various muscles and nerves to signals from the brain. Nerve Conduction tests are used to evaluate whether or not a nerve stimulated by electricity transmits these signals and at what speed.

The functions of the spinal cord and nerves are monitored for safety by Somatosensory Evoked Potentials, **SSEP,** and Motor Evoked Potentials, **MEP**, during surgical procedures to decompress, correct, and stabilize the spine.

Various blood tests are of value in evaluating patients with spine complaints. These can include blood tests for infection (sedimentation rate, white blood cell count, and blood cultures) as well as bone and tissue samples. Patients with arthritis are tested for rheumatoid arthritis, systemic lupus erythematosus, gout, ankylosing spondylitis, and other diseases with indicators found in the blood. Samples of spinal fluid are analyzed for cells indicative of infection, tumor or trauma.

Chapter 3. Non-Surgical Options in Neck Care

Prior to considering any surgical procedure, it is wise to pursue appropriate non-surgical therapy. Most surgeons recommend a three to six-month course of non-surgical treatments prior to spine surgery.

John, a forty-year-old accountant, awoke on Monday morning with a very stiff neck following a weekend of doing yard work that included pruning large bushes, digging, and raking. He had a hard time finding a comfortable sleep position due to his neck pain. Turning and bending his neck was painful due to spasm of his neck muscles.

Most likely, John has strained muscles and ligaments that support the vertebrae in his neck. A few days of rest, ice packs, and over-the-counter medication such as Motrin®, Aleve®, or Tylenol® will usually resolve the problem. Stretching prior to doing the yard work and using good body mechanics may have prevented this.

It is estimated that during one's lifetime, most of us will have one or more episodes of a stiff neck. Often these occur without any obvious cause. John, who has a sedentary job, the cause of his acute neck pain was probably due to his "not being in shape" to tackle the rigors of a weekend of yard work.

If your neck pain causes you difficulty with your normal activities, what can you do to aid your recovery?

Following an acute injury to your neck, ice applied to the painful area can reduce swelling and pain. Short periods of bed rest and a reduction in stressful physical activity may accelerate recovery. A soft cervical collar to give added support to your neck may also help.

Non-steroidal anti-inflammatories drugs, **NSAIDs**, are often effective in reducing pain and improving motion and function. Ibuprofen, naproxen, and diclofenac are effective in alleviating inflammatory conditions of the spine joints and tendons. Although serious side effects are rare, gastrointestinal bleeding, fluid retention, kidney damage, and cardiac failure may occur with the use of **high** and **prolonged** doses of NSAIDs. Some **topical anti-inflammatory solutions and gels** are available by prescription and can be effective. Narcotics such as codeine, hydrocodone and oxycodone may be used for short-term pain control following injury and surgery. Long-term use results in dependence and addiction. Muscle relaxants may be of some value in the early phases of acute neck pain to reduce muscle spasms. Neurontin®, Gabapentin, and Tramadol may also be useful.

Cortisone was discovered by Phillip Hench and Edward Kendall of the Mayo Clinic when they noted that during pregnancy some patients with rheumatoid arthritis got better and several went into remission. This was due to higher than normal levels of cortisol produced during pregnancy. In the late 1940s, cortisone, a steroid drug, became available. Short courses of oral steroids, such as Prednisone® and Medrol®, can be very effective in reducing nerve root and inflammation-generated pain. However, these medications do not result in any reversal of the arthritic process, which continues on.

Injection of various types of cortisone in conjunction with local anesthetics into inflamed and arthritic joints has brought relief to many patients by disrupting the inflammatory cycle of pain. Patients with suspected infection and those on anticoagulants are not candidates for these types of injections. If needed, these injections can be given every four to six months.

Platelet Rich Plasma (**PRP**) collected from the patient's blood and stem cells harvested from fat and bone marrow injected into painful joints of the spine may reduce pain and improve function. Although biologic approaches to treating back pain are gaining popularity, results are variable. Long-term outcomes from this type of treatment are not available.

Epidural steroid injections (**ESI**) are placed into the spinal canal outside the protective dura, the sheath surrounding the spinal cord and its nerves, to reduce nerve-root-generated pain. Several types of targeted nerve root blocks are used to determine which nerves are responsible for generating the pain. After injection of a local anesthetic around the affected nerve root, the patient is asked if their usual pain level is less or abated. The addition of cortisone to the diagnostic block may reduce the nerve-generated pain for variable periods of time. These diagnostic nerve root blocks done by skilled physicians specializing in Pain Management using X-Ray guidance are extremely helpful in directing surgical treatment to the exact anatomical areas responsible for the patient's pain. For facet joint mediated pain, anesthetic blocks are done on the small nerves that supply these joints. If the patient has relief of pain from the blocks, there are techniques to destroy these nerves, **ablation.**

Transcutaneous electrical nerve stimulators, *TENS*, are sometimes helpful in overriding and masking painful stimuli. These devices are applied to the skin around the painful area, and the patient adjusts the intensity and frequency of the current. A device called a **dorsal column stimulator** can be helpful in managing patients with chronic pain due to various spinal disorders and following spinal surgery. The dorsal column stimulator is placed through a small incision into the spinal canal on the back surface of the dura. The generator is attached to the stimulator wires and is tested for effectiveness in reducing pain prior to its permanent implantation in the body. Pain Management physicians provide care for patients requiring further pain control with medications and injections following surgery.

Physical and occupational therapy can be effective in treating acute and chronic pain. Stretching, strength training, and supportive bracing under the supervision of a skilled therapist can be very helpful during the acute onset of a painful spine condition, as well as during rehabilitation following surgery and trauma. Traction applied to the neck is often helpful in relieving pain. It can be applied by using weights and pulleys or by machines. This can be done at home using a neck harness that fits around your neck and base of your head. The halter is hooked up to weights to provide a vertical steady pull to relax and stretch tight muscles.

Overhead Cervical Traction Apparatus

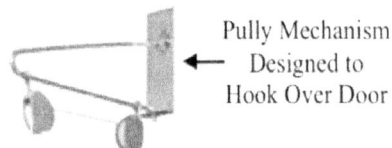

Pully Mechanism
Designed to
Hook Over Door

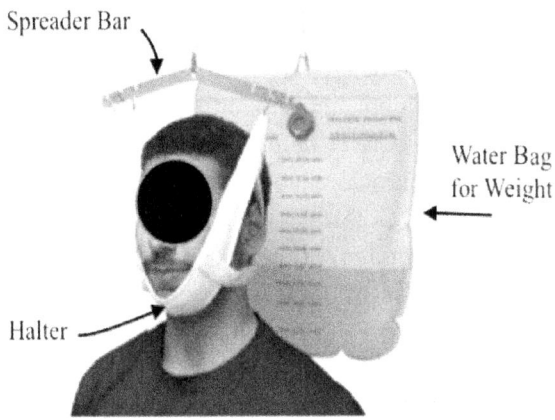

Spreader Bar

Water Bag
for Weight

Halter

If your joints are not stretched to their limits on a regular basis, the amount of motion they will allow will diminish. We all lose some range of motion as we age, but we can counteract that somewhat and even improve our range of motion through stretching.

Muscle strength training is important if you want to maintain function and agility in performing your routine daily activities without overloading and fatiguing the muscles that control the movement and alignment of your spine. Often the major muscles of your cervical spine get lazy and need reinforcement by doing strengthening exercises such as bringing your neck forward, backward and to the side using your hands for counter resistance.

Many of you have been to chiropractors for neck and back pain. Most of these practitioners are trained in providing non-operative care. Be sure you have had an adequate evaluation and diagnosis before undergoing treatment.

We recommend seeing a medical doctor spine specialist if you have neurologic symptoms such as loss of feeling or weakness in your arms or legs or if your pain persists despite chiropractic treatment.

Some Self-Help Tips

Attorney Bob spent many work hours at his computer. He had never had a neck injury, but he had noticed over the years that his ability to rotate his neck was diminishing. He even learned that he could not drink liquids from a can very well. He could not tilt his head back far enough to empty the can. Over time he began to have pain running down his right arm and intermittent tingling in his fingers when working for long periods.

His orthopaedic surgeon confirmed that he had generalized degeneration of his discs and arthritis of his cervical spine. He had no detectable weakness or loss of sensation, but his neck motion was significantly limited.

Questioning revealed that he, like many seniors, wore bifocal eyeglasses. His surgeon suggested that he have his eye doctor give him a prescription for eyeglasses just for computer work. They would give him clear vision to read from his computer screen without having to lean forward and tilt his head backwards to bring the bifocals into play. The glasses would not work for reading papers or distance seeing, but would be ideal for reading from a computer. Bob embraced the idea and his arm pain and tingling were resolved. In fact, at a visit to his dentist six months later, the dentist, also a senior, complained of arm pain and tingling. Bob told him about his eyeglasses and "cured" him, too. Having an extra set of eyeglasses may be a bit inconvenient, but both of these professional men happily chose that over spine surgery.

Another way we can help ourselves is observing how we sit. This is especially noticeable when driving for long distances. If the seat back is straight up, after a while we tend to slump down and forward. In order to keep our head erect we have to tilt back at the neck, which reduces the openings in the back of the spine where the nerve roots exit. Simply tilting the seat back a few degrees can work wonders.

If your neck is stiff, you may find that riding bicycles gives you problems. If so, be sure you are not leaning forward too much, as this requires you to hyperextend your neck to see where you are going.

Have you been told to swim for exercise but you cannot turn your neck enough to breath while doing so? Try swimming with a mask and a snorkel.

Chapter 4: Common Disorders Affecting the Neck

"Pinched nerves," *cervical radiculopathy,* due to herniated disc and cervical disc disease are common disorders, which may affect your neck.

Pain around the shoulder, arm, and hand may be caused by irritation or compression of one or more of the cervical nerve roots.
In most patients, the symptoms are of short duration and resolve without treatment.

If a nerve is irritated, *radiculitis* results **without loss** of motor, reflex, or sensory function. When a nerve is compressed or a nerve has disease within its structure, *radiculopathy* results. **Loss of muscle function, sensation, and reflex changes are seen with radiculopathy, but not with radiculitis.**

Degenerative disc disease starts in the third decade of life. The discs between our vertebrae become less supple and begin to wear out. This is due to loss of hydration of the nucleus and the occurrence of tears and fissures in the outer casing, *the annulus fibrosus.* Nuclear material can escape through these tears and fissures. In an attempt by the body to stabilize the failing disc, bone spurs, *osteophytes,* are formed along the surfaces of the vertebrae, the facet joints and the connecting Luscha joints. As the disc losses height, the space for the spinal cord and nerve roots become diminished.

Progression and Effects of Degenerative Disc Disease

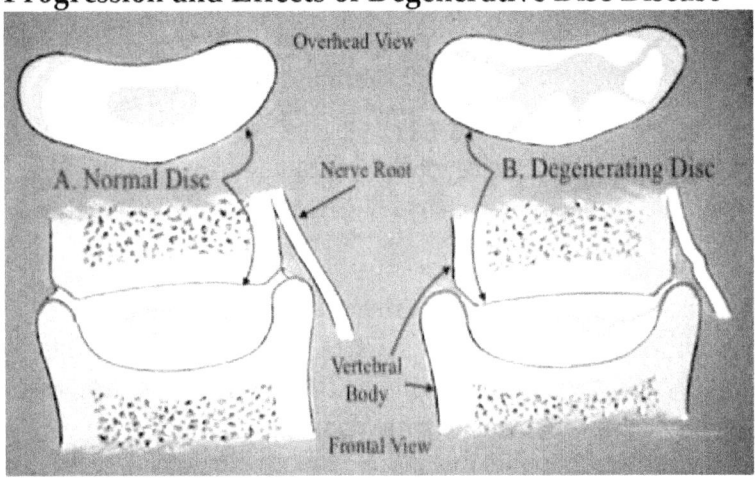

A. Normal disc
B. Degenerating disc with loss of nuclear material and fissures in annulus fibrosus

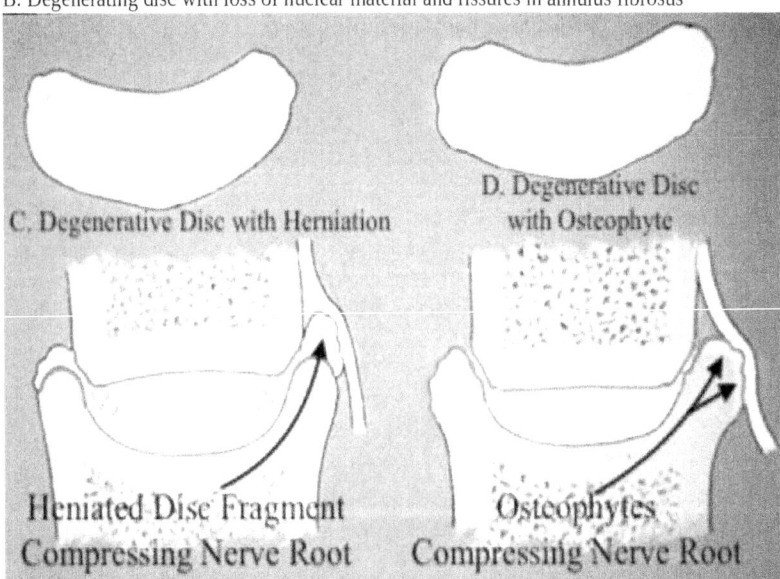

C. Degenerative disc with herniation resulting in nerve root compression

D. Degenerative disc with osteophytes resulting in nerve root compression

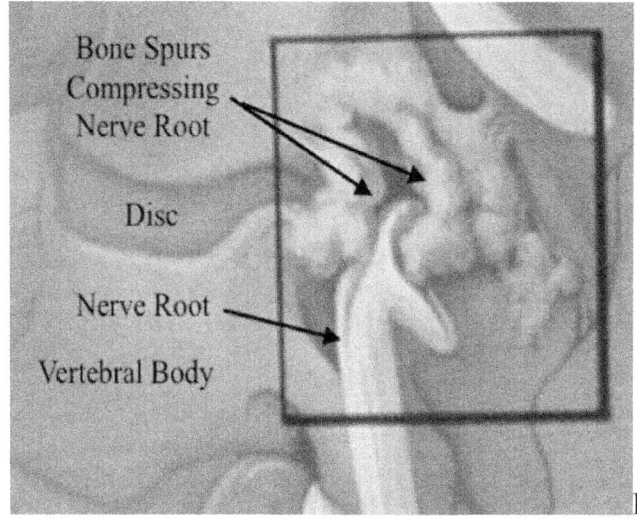

Bone spurs, *osteophytes*, in the facet joints and Luscha joints eventually result in compression of the nerve roots as they exit through the foramen, *foramenal stenosis*, and those that cause constriction of the neural canal result in impingement on the spinal cord, *spinal stenosis*.

Four out of five people over age 55 will show X-ray changes of deteriorated cervical discs at one or more locations. Nearly fifty percent will experience one attack of neck pain with radiation into the arm, forearm, or hand. About a third of patients with persistent and prolonged radiating pain may require surgical treatment.

Clinical Presentation:

The occurrence of cervical nerve root compression is often insidious without antecedent injury. The pain may be intense, of long or short duration, and may interfere with sleep. Avoiding activities, which place the neck in extension and lateral bending, may lessen symptoms. Putting the affected arm behind the head will relieve tension on the involved nerve roots.

Limited motion of the neck is common, especially extension, rotation, and side bending. Radiating pain is often intensified in the extremity when the examiner places the neck in extension and toward the symptomatic side, the

Spurling's test.

Radiculopathy Nerve Patterns

- With a C5 radiculopathy, there is pain around the shoulder blade and weakness of the rotator cuff and deltoid shoulder muscles.
- With a C6 radiculopathy, there is weakness of the biceps and wrist extensors, a diminished biceps reflex and numbness of the thumb and index finger.
- With a C7 radiculopathy there is weakness of the triceps, finger extensors and wrist flexors muscles and a depressed triceps reflex with numbness of the long finger.
- With a C8 radiculopathy there is weakness of the small muscles of the hand and numbness in the ring and little fingers.

Larry, a 55-year-old financial advisor, had a gradual onset of neck and right arm pain. He noted some numbness of his right thumb and index finger and weakness of his wrist. He got some relief with NSAIDs. After a series of X-rays, his primary care physician recommended a course of physical therapy and traction, which gave him some relief. However, the numbness and weakness persisted, and he had difficulty sleeping because of nagging arm pain. An MRI showed compression of the C6 nerve root due to a degenerative disc and bone spurs in close proximity to the nerve root. A block of the C6 nerve was done with a local anesthetic. He had complete relief of his pain until the nerve block wore off. Larry elected to have the degenerative disc and bone spurs removed and an anterior cervical fusion using bone from a bone bank. He did well following surgery and had return of sensation and muscle strength.

Compression of the nerve root results in pain and varying degrees of sensory and motor weakness. This process may occur at one or more levels, the most common being in the discs between the fourth, fifth and sixth cervical vertebra.

Treatment with NSAIDs, a short course of oral cortisone, muscle relaxants and physical therapy is successful in over two-thirds of patients affected with degenerative cervical disc disease. In those patients with compression of a nerve root with sensory and muscle loss, surgery may be necessary.

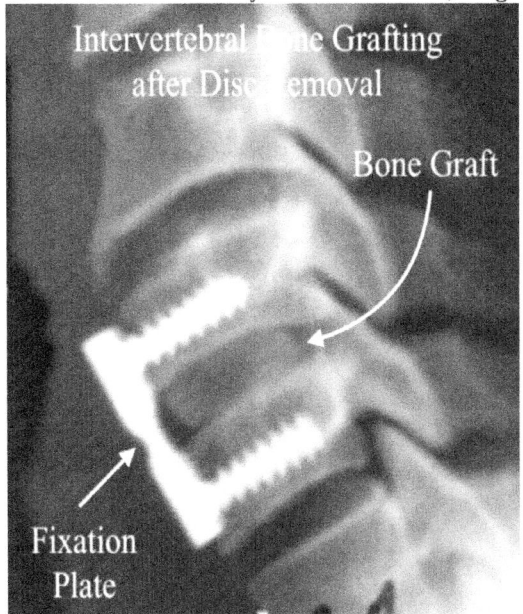

Intervertebral Bone Grafting after Disc Removal

Bone Graft

Fixation Plate

The most successful surgical treatment during the last 60 years has been removal of the offending disc and decompression of the affected nerve root. This is accomplished by approaching the affected level from the front of the spine through a small incision in the neck. After removing the degenerative disc and spurs, a bone graft is placed between the vertebrae to restore vertical height to the collapsed disc space. This results in an indirect decompression of the nerve roots due to widening and opening of the nerve root canals. In order to prevent displacement of the graft and to stabilize it during the healing process, a plate is applied with screws.

The most common complaints after this type of surgery are sore throat, difficulty swallowing, and hoarseness due to swelling and irritation of the throat, esophagus, and vocal cords. These usually resolve a few days after surgery. On occasion, the nerve root will be slow to recover due to being manipulated during surgery. Healing of the fusion is rarely a problem. Permanent damage to the nerve root or spinal cord is extremely rare.

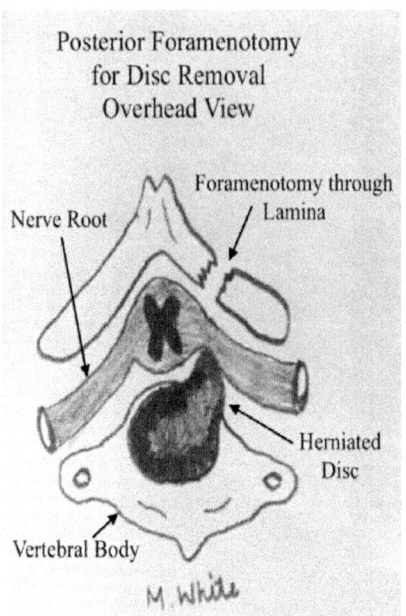

Posterior Foramenotomy
for Disc Removal
Overhead View

Nerve Root

Foramenotomy through
Lamina

Herniated
Disc

Vertebral Body

M. White

Another approach is to decompress the nerve root though a small incision on the back of the neck.This is refered to as a *posterior foramenotomy* and *discectomy* where the offending bone and disc compressing the nerve root are removed to provide room for the nerve root. This procedure has a high success rate. As with the anterior cervical fusion, nerve root recovery may be delayed due to manipulation of the nerve root.

Posterior Foramenotomy
for Disc Removal

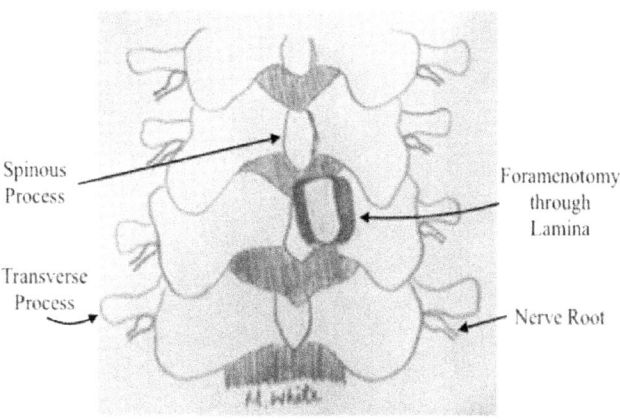

Spinous Process

Foramenotomy through Lamina

Transverse Process

Nerve Root

Posterior View

In younger patients with one or two discs that need surgical treatment, a cervical disc replacement is an option. This is done though a small incision in the front of the neck. After the disc is removed, the surfaces of the vertebrae are prepared for placement of the cervical disc implant. The ten-plus year outcomes are showing good results in a significant number of patients with a low rate of revision or the need for additional surgery at adjacent levels.

Artificial Cervical Disc

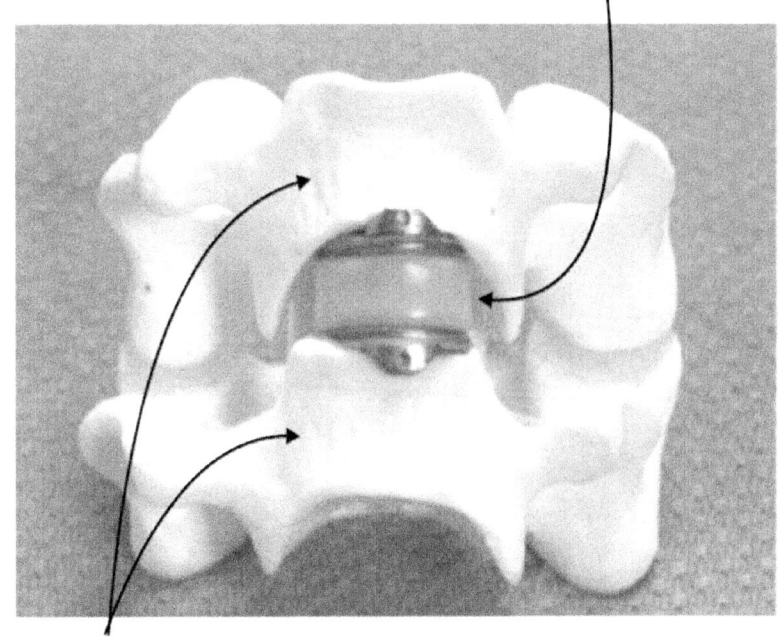

Vertebral Bodies   Frontal View

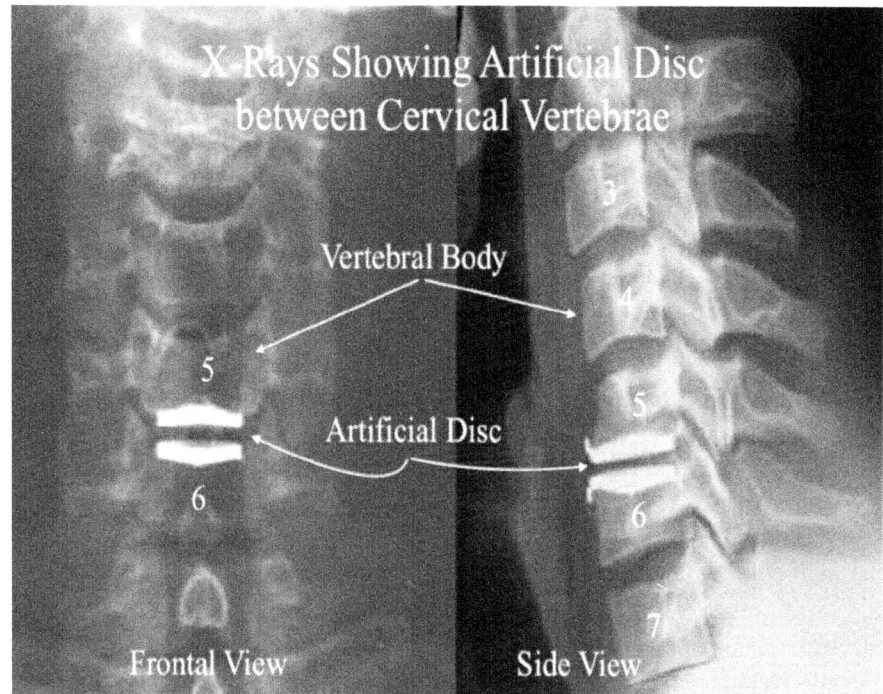

X-Rays Showing Artificial Disc between Cervical Vertebrae

Vertebral Body

Artificial Disc

Frontal View

Side View

Cervical Ribs

Cervical ribs are usually bilateral, *on both sides of the spine*, and may cause compression on the C8 root between the first chest rib and the extra cervical rib just above it. Those affected complain of pain and tingling in the arm and the ring and little fingers. Compression of the axillary artery and vein may occur with a cervical rib causing pain and swelling with poor blood supply in the affected extremity.

Syringomyelia

Some patients form fluid-filled cysts within the tissue of the spinal cord from increased pressure from their own spinal fluid. This results in a condition called *syringomyelia*. Patients may experience radiating pain, weakness, loss of balance, and dexterity in the extremities. Decompression, drainage and shunting procedures are used to relieve pressure and restore the flow of cerebral spinal fluid. Patients with demyelinating diseases such *as multiple sclerosis* often also experience radiating pain.

Cervical Cord Compression, Cervical Stenosis, Cervical Myelopathy

Hector, a 69-year-old retired auto mechanic, noted difficulty with walking, balance and with fine motor tasks using his hands such as buttoning up his shirt. On occasion, when flexing his neck, he would have "sharp pains going down his spine." He was also having urgency to urinate. A neurologist found that he had weakness of the small muscles of his hands and extremely hyperactive, abnormal reflexes. X-rays of his neck confirmed extensive arthritis. An MRI showed marked narrowing of the spinal canal due to degeneration of the discs and extensive bone spurs, which were compressing the spinal cord and nerve roots. He was treated with medication and physical therapy, but he did not improve. Surgery was done to take pressure off his spinal cord. This involved removal of bone from the back part of his spine and widening of his spinal canal by a procedure called *laminoplasty*. After the surgery, he had improvement in his walking, balance, and use of his hands.

Cervical cord compression, *cervical myelopathy*, occurs in older individuals and is progressive in the majority of those affected. The internal area of the cervical spinal canal decreases due to narrowing of the discs and formation of arthritic facets and connecting joints, *cervical stenosis*. This results in compression of the spinal cord and nerve roots, *myelopathy and radiculopathy*.

Patients will experience difficulty, as Hector did, with simple tasks like buttoning his shirt and picking up small objects such as coins due to weakness of the small muscles that motor the fingers and thumbs. Because of the increased muscle tone and hyperactive reflexes, balance is altered, which may result in frequent falls. Flexion of the neck further reduces the diameter of the spinal canal and results in irritation of the sensory portion of the spinal cord. This causes intermittent sharp pain traveling down the spine.
MRI will show the extent and degree of spinal cord and nerve root compression. In those patients who cannot undergo an MRI, a myelogram and CT scan will clarify the diagnosis. The most common areas affected are at the third, fourth, fifth, sixth and seventh cervical vertebrae. In two-thirds of those with cervical myelopathy, the disease will progress if not treated. Medication, rest, and neck immobilization may provide some temporary relief.

In order to take pressure off the spinal cord and nerve roots, bone is removed from the back of the spine, *cervical laminectomy*. This procedure is done at multiple levels to decompress the spinal cord and nerve roots.

Cervical Laminectomy
Exposing the Dura Mater

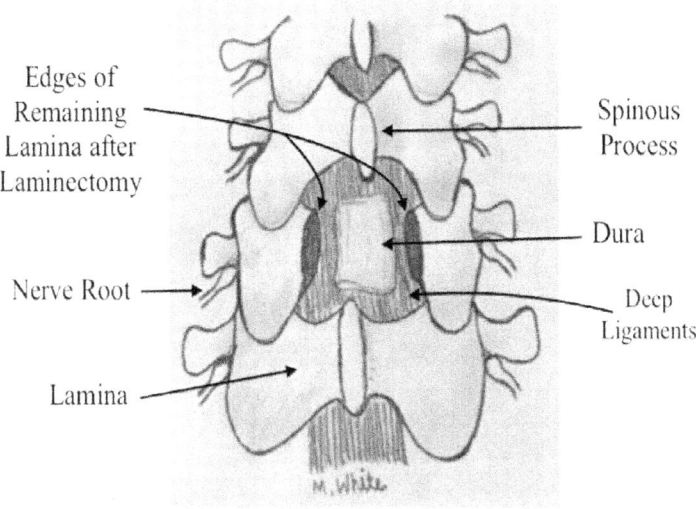

Edges of Remaining Lamina after Laminectomy

Nerve Root

Lamina

Spinous Process

Dura

Deep Ligaments

M. White

Posterior View

Another method of dealing with the compression is to enlarge the spinal canal to provide more space for the spinal cord and nerve roots. This can be done by removing bone from the laminae to open and expand the spinal canal, *cervical laminoplasty*. It is usually done at multiple levels. Pieces of bone are inserted to maintain the expansion. These procedures are quite delicate and are performed with spinal cord monitoring.

Compressed Spinal Cord
due to Narrowed
Spinal Canal

Laminoplasty, Step 1.
Removal of Wedge
of Bone

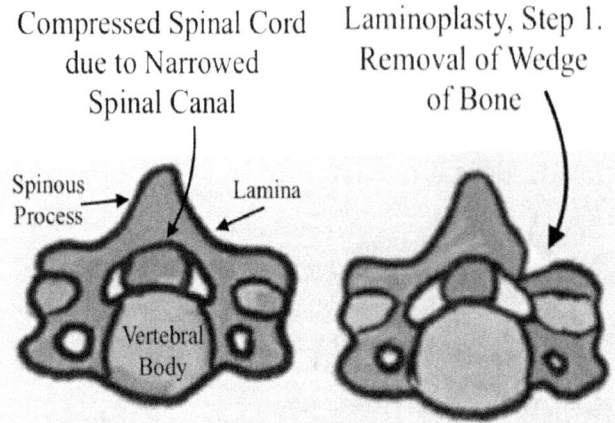

Spinous
Process

Lamina

Vertebral
Body

Laminoplasty, Step 3.
Bone Graft Secured
into Place with
Plate and Screws

Laminoplasty, Step 2.
Bone Cut on Opposite Side
to Allow Enlarging
the Spinal Canal

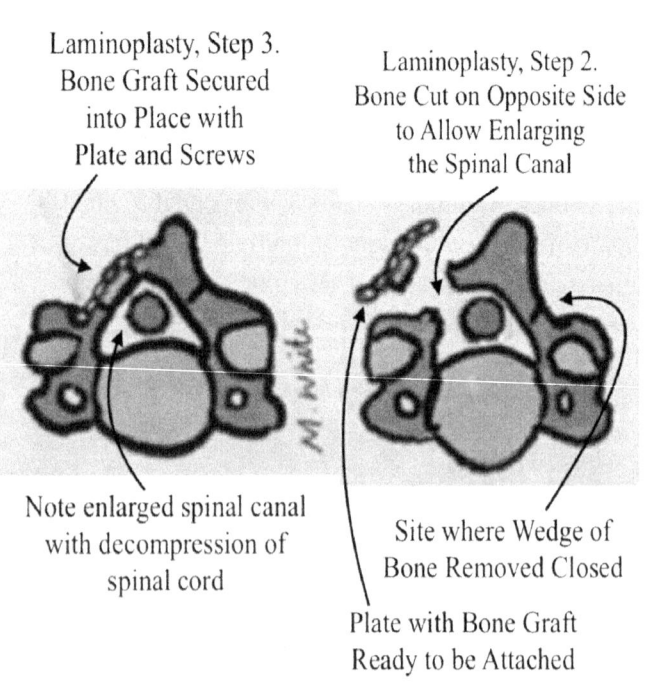

Note enlarged spinal canal
with decompression of
spinal cord

Site where Wedge of
Bone Removed Closed

Plate with Bone Graft
Ready to be Attached

Complications may include bleeding, collections of blood around the spinal cord following surgery that require drainage to remove pressure on the spinal cord and temporary loss of nerve root function. Improvement of walking, balance, and fine motor control may take several months. Results are good in those patients who have been operated on within 12-24 months after the onset of their symptoms. Results of surgery are not good in patients with more severe and progressive cervical myelopathy of longer duration.

Another commonly used surgical approach to treat cervical myelopathy is to remove the degenerative discs and adjacent bone from the front of the spine and to replace these areas with spacers and bone grafts. This results in removal of pressure on the spinal cord and restoration of the spinal canal length and area through fusion. On occasion it may be necessary to do both front and back surgery to relieve the compression.

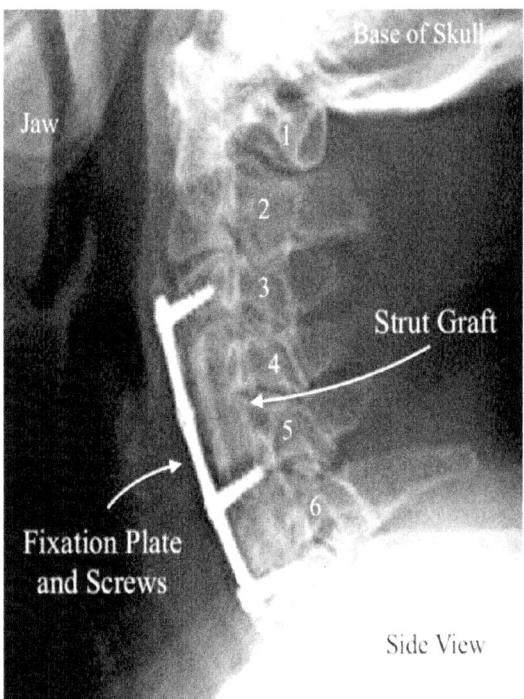

Cervical Spine Following Multiple Level Anterior
Decompression and Fusion for Myelopathy

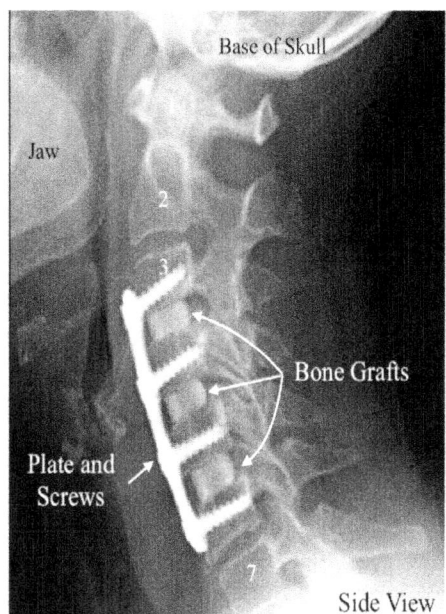

Cervical Spine Following Multi-level Decompression
and Fusion with Multiple Bone Grafts and Plate

Chapter 5: Arthritis, Cancer, Infections, and Fractures

Arthritis of the Cervical Spine

Rheumatoid arthritis may severely affect the upper end of the cervical spine due to the unique anatomy of the connection between the skull and the first and second cervical vertebrae. The disease causes erosion of the ligaments and joints between the skull, *occiput*, and the first two cervical vertebrae, *C1 and C2*. This destructive process results in neck pain due to instability. Today, there are several biologic immunotherapy medications such as Humira® which can halt the progression of rheumatoid arthritis. However, in some patients, surgical stabilization of the occiput, C1 and C2 vertebrae is necessary to improve function and relieve pain.

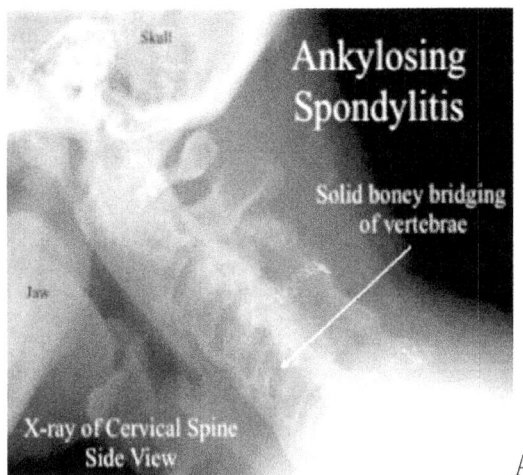

A condition called ankylosing spondylitis, **AS**, is a type of inflammatory arthritis that leads to progressive stiffness and fusion of the movable parts of the spine, the hips, sacroiliac joints, and shoulders. AS, makes one prone to spinal fractures due to lack of mobility and fragility of the vertebral bone. Patients with AS test positive for the HLA-B 27 antigen. There are several biologic immunotherapy medications being used to treat psoriatic arthritis, arthritis due to inflammatory bowel diseases, and AS.

Some patients with AS require surgery to correct what is called a chin on chest deformity. The neck fuses in a position of flexion making it difficult for the patient to look forward. To correct this deformity, the bone at the base of the cervical spine is removed to allow for repositioning of the neck in a more normal position so that the patient can look straight ahead.

Surgical Correction of Ankylosing Spondylitis

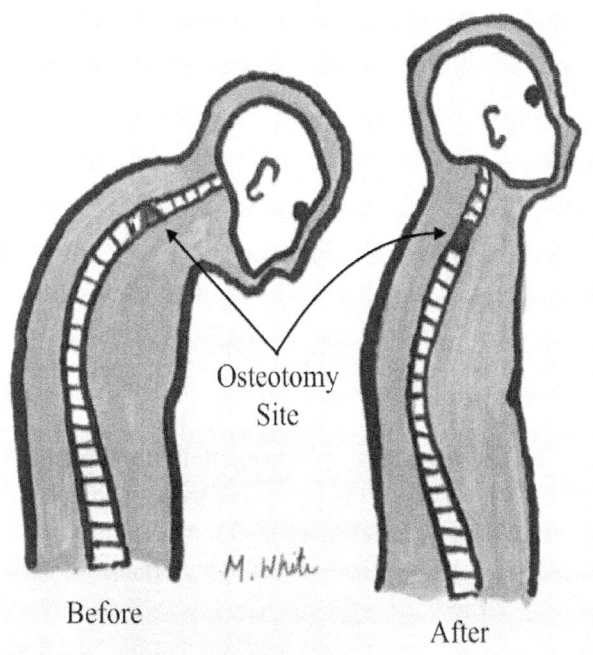

Osteotomy
Site

M. White

Before

After

Cancer of the Cervical Spine

Metastatic cancer, cancer arising in one place and migrating to other places, frequently finds a home in the marrow of our long bones and spine. About 20,000 patients each year have cancer metastases to their spine. Lung, breast, prostate, and kidney tumors are common sources of cancer metastasizing to the spine.

Ginny, age 55, requested consultation about persistent pain in her neck, worse at night and when she was inactive. Imaging studies showed two large bony tumors in her cervical vertebrae. She had had cancer of her breast treated several years ago. A biopsy confirmed that these were due to metastatic cancer from the breast. She underwent radiation and chemotherapy treatments, which were successful.

Much less frequent, are primary bone tumors that have their origin in bone. Some are benign bony growths like *osteochondromas*, and others are malignant and life threatening such as *osteosarcoma*, bone cancer, and *chondrosarcoma*, cartilage cancer. These are very aggressive and invasive. These cancers present with deep unrelenting pain not related to movement or change in position. Pain at night is one of the hallmarks alerting the doctor to be concerned that this complaint needs attention. In addition to pain, the patient might experience progressive loss of motor and sensory function if the tumor causes pressure on adjacent nerves or the spinal cord. Fracture of the involved bone may occur without trauma.

Chordomas, tumors of cartilage, are malignant tumors of the spine. They commonly occur at the base of the brainstem and in the upper cervical spine in youngsters and in the sacrum during the 5th to 7th decade of life. A combination of surgery and various types of radiotherapy are used to treat them. Imatinib®, an immunotherapy drug has been helpful in suppressing tumor growth.

Giant cell tumors are aggressive destructive tumors that destroy bone in young females. Because of the vascularity of the tumor preoperative blockage of the feeder blood vessels is done prior to surgical resection. Denosumab®, has been used recently in treating patients with non-resectable tumors and in those with recurrence following surgery.

Our bone marrow is full of many types of cells, including red and white blood cells, lymphocytes, platelets, plasma cells, *osteoblasts*, bone forming cells, *osteoclasts*, bone destroying cells, and an array of *stem cells*. Stem cells are the source and generators of our specialized blood and tissue cells. When any of these cells multiply out of control, malignant cells are produced.

Multiple myeloma is a cancer of plasma cells, which originate in bone and is associated with pain and spontaneous fractures. The presence of abnormal antibodies in the blood and urine, Bence-Jones paraproteins and a positive needle biopsy confirm the diagnosis. The treating physician should be suspicious of multiple myeloma in a patient with one or more compression fractures of the spine. MRI and CT scans are used to evaluate the location, type, and extent of the disease. The abnormal myeloma proteins in the urine deposit casts, which block kidney function and result in renal failure. Chemotherapy is used to eradicate the cancerous plasma cells. If the patient has a good response to chemotherapy with a significant reduction of the abnormal plasma cells, *a stem cell transfer* using the patient's own bone marrow may result in remission.

Various types of leukemia due to abnormal white cells, such as *myelocytic* and *lymphocytic,* may result in pain, anemia, fever, and frequent infections due to a diseased and altered immune system. Chemotherapy and radiation are effective in suppressing leukemia. Fractures may occur in bone weakened by infiltration of leukemia cells.

Infiltration of destructive cancer cells can cause sudden collapse of one or more vertebrae, instability of that segment of the spine and compression of the spinal cord. Depending on the location of the spinal cord compression, loss of function in the lower extremities, *paraplegia* or loss of function in both the upper and lower extremities, *quadriplegia* may result.

Metastatic lesions to the spine are best treated with chemotherapy and, in some cases, targeted immunotherapy. Metastatic cancer from the breast, lungs, prostate, kidney, and gastrointestinal tract tumors respond to radiation therapy. Surgery may be an option for patients expected to live a number of months and in relatively stable health. Chemotherapy and radiation are often used to reduce tumor size prior to surgical intervention. Imaging studies are utilized to evaluate whether or not the tumor is amenable to surgical resection. Total resection of the diseased vertebra with preservation of the spinal cord and reconstruction with bone grafts, implants, and metallic fixation is feasible. Complications following this type of surgery may be serious and outcomes may be disappointing.

Cervical nerve root tumors, which are called *neurofibromas,* can cause radiating pain. Multiple neurofibromas, *neurofibromatosis,* may affect multiple nerve roots. These erode into the bone around the cervical foramen as they enlarge and cause compression of the affected nerve roots. The disease can also cause spinal deformity, for example, the posture of the **Hunchback of Notre Dame.**

Pancoast tumor is a malignant tumor of the lung, which grows into the cervical nerve roots where they join together under the collarbone. The tumor causes severe pain and weakness in the involved shoulder, arm, and hand.

Infections of the Spine

Henry, a healthy 30-year-old, was recovering at home after undergoing a cervical discectomy, when he had a sudden chill followed by a fever of 103 degrees. He also had increasing pain in the area of his neck surgery. He reported this to his surgeon, who admitted him to the hospital. Blood tests and cultures confirmed that Henry was suffering from a postoperative infection. He received intravenous antibiotics, which were targeted to eradicate his type of infection, and he recovered.

Joe, an adult onset diabetic, had surgery for cervical spinal stenosis. A few days later, he felt poorly and had a low-grade fever with increasing pain in his operative area. He had received antibiotics before and for a day following surgery. Drainage from his incision was sent to the laboratory for culture, which grew "staph." Antibiotics were restarted and he was returned to the operating room for drainage of a large abscess involving the tissues in the area of his surgery. After several weeks, the infection was brought under control, and he returned home.

When surgical site infection occurs, we consider these factors:

1. Host resistance
2. Inoculum
3. Virulence of the bacteria
4. Presence of a foreign body

By "Host Resistance," we mean the ability of the body to resist infection. Our skin is covered, and our intestines are filled with trillions of bacteria, our "biome." Every time we brush our teeth, we send bacteria into our blood stream, generally to no effect. If your resistance is diminished by A.I.D.S, *autoimmune disease syndrome*, diabetes or chronic use of steroids, you stand an increased chance of infection from surgery.

The rate of infection following spine surgery increases tenfold if your diabetes is in poor control. Your blood glucose needs to be in a suitable range before, during and after surgery.

The "Inoculum" is the number of bacteria that gets into the host's bloodstream. A tiny amount such as what we may get from brushing our teeth is unlikely to cause problems, but a huge amount is likely to overwhelm any host.

Surgeons do all they can to avoid this by extensively scrubbing their hands, wearing sterile clothing and gloves along with shields to protect their patients from surgeon-generated particles. Procedures, such as, sterilizing instruments, using soaps and antiseptics to prepare the patient's skin, and establishing a "sterile field" around the incision and managing airflow in the operating room are done to decrease infections. Preventing infection is always on the minds of all operating room personnel who monitor each other on behalf of the patient.

Likewise, patients need to carefully prepare their own bodies by thoroughly washing with appropriate soaps before surgery. They should avoid skin cuts and scratches, especially on or near the body part having the surgery.

For spine surgery where implants are inserted into the body, we recommend getting dental work and regular dental cleaning well in advance of surgery.

The nose harbors bacteria that could infect the host. We recommend using nasal swabs for MRSA, *methicillin resistant staphylococcus aureus*, a particularly difficult bacteria to eradicate. If MRSA is found in the nose, it can be treated before surgery with a specific antibiotic ointment.

"Virulence" describes the inherent aggressiveness of the bacteria. Highly virulent bacteria are very aggressive, so a smaller dose can cause an infection that may not occur with less virulent bacteria.

We live with low-virulence bacteria all of the time, but when the bad boys, the highly virulent ones, come along we are apt to be in trouble.

A subtopic about virulence is the susceptibility of bacteria to antibiotics. Some, such as MRSA and others, are less susceptible to the usual antibiotics than others. They have become resistant over time from exposure to commonly used antibiotics.

Penicillin was the first antibiotic. Over time many bacteria became "penicillin resistant." Methicillin was developed to fight penicillin- resistant bacteria, but ultimately bacteria developed resistance to it. As we have regularly used the stronger, more-toxic-to-human antibiotics, some bacteria have become resistant to them, too.

We need to be judicious in our use of antibiotics, because bacteria are constantly evolving and developing resistance. Our scientists are diligently developing new antibiotics, but it is a formidable task that we only make more challenging by overusing the ones that we have.

An important point for the short term is that surgeons prophylactically use broad-spectrum antibiotics beginning just before surgery and then for only a dose or two more. The idea is to help knock out any bacteria that may get into the surgical wound. That has been scientifically demonstrated to reduce the incidence of wound infection.

A "Foreign Body" is anything in the body that we were not born with. It is well known that the presence of a foreign body like a spinal implant makes eradication of infection more difficult. Since spinal implants are used to stabilize the spine, they are usually retained when the wound is reopened, and infected soft tissue is removed to treat infection.

Spinal infections may occur in patients with diabetes, those on long-term cortisone therapy, those with H.I.V., and in patients who are immunocompromised by diseases and medications that reduce a person's immunity. The most common complaints are neck and back pain that is constant and worse at night. There may be stiffness and reduced spinal motion. Typically, an infection is carried in the blood stream to the spine from an infected organ such as skin, lung or kidney.

Blood tests, cultures of blood and drainage fluids, bone scan, CT scans, and MRI are helpful in diagnosing and managing spinal infection.

It is important to **contact your physician** if you think you have an infection. **Do not start yourself on some random antibiotic** that you have saved in your medicine cabinet. Even antibiotics that are not effective against the causative bacteria can interfere with laboratory cultures and delay treatment with the proper, targeted antibiotic. Taking a random antibiotic will also convert one's biome from bacteria that are less resistant to antibiotics to ones that are more resistant, so if an infection occurs it will be more difficult to treat.

If an abscess develops in the space surrounding the spinal cord, *epidural abscess*, the patient may experience extremity weakness, numbness and lack of bladder and bowel control, *incontinence*. It is imperative to remove the epidural abscess to preserve spinal cord function. An infection that invades bone may result in progressive bone destruction and instability of the spine segment, which can also lead to permanent loss of spinal cord function and paralysis. Prolonged targeted antibiotics to combat sepsis coupled with

Glossary

Arthritis: an inflamed joint

Osteoarthritis: affects *multiple* joints during aging. Bone spurs, *osteophytes*, occur. The joint space narrows due to loss of articular cartilage.

Degenerative Arthritis: *affects one or a few joints.* It is similar to osteoarthritis as regards symptoms and findings on imaging studies.

Post-traumatic Arthritis: results from damage to the joint following fracture and injury

Gout: type of inflammatory arthritis due to uric acid crystals deposition in the joint

Pseudogout type of inflammatory arthritis due to pyrophosphate crystals deposition in the joint

Inflammatory Arthritis: caused by one's own immune system attack against the body

Reiter's disease: inflammatory "reactive" arthritis and conjunctivitis, which may affect the urinary, gastrointestinal, pulmonary, and genital organs.

Rheumatoid arthritis: autoimmune disease that attacks the joint's lining, *synovium* and releases enzymes that damage the articular cartilage and weaken the underlying bone

Systemic Lupus Erythematosus: autoimmune disease that attacks the joints, kidneys, skin and multiple other organs

Psoriatic Arthritis: autoimmune disease that affects the skin and joints

Anatomic Parts and Positions

Anterior, Ventral, the front of the spine

Posterior, Dorsal, the back view of the spine

Lateral, the side view of the spine

Cranial, Superior, toward the head

Caudal, Inferior, toward the tail end of the spine

Flexion, forward bending of the spine

Extension, backward bending of the spine

Rotation, turning or twisting of the spine

Lateral, bending to the side

Lordosis, normal forward curve of the cervical and lumbar spine segments

Kyphosis, normal backward curve of the thoracic spine segment

Scoliosis, combination of lateral bending and rotation of the spine

Spondylolistheses, forward slip of one vertebra upon another

Cranium, skull

Occiput, the back, lower portion of the skull

Vertebral body, a cylindrical bone that forms the base of the spinal canal

Pedicles, projections extending from the lateral aspects of the back of the vertebral body connecting it to the laminae and helping form the spinal canal

Laminae, plates of bone covering the back of the spinal canal

Spinous process, projections of bone you can feel on the back of your neck

Superior and Inferior facets, joint surfaces that allow for coupling of one vertebra to the other

Transverse process, lateral projections that provide for muscle attachments

Spinal Canal, the mostly round, bony canal formed by the back of the vertebral body, the pedicles and the laminae that provides protection for the spinal cord and nerves

Intervertebral Disc, the gel-like material, the *nucleus pulposus*, surrounded by interlacing fibers of the annulus fibrosus with attachments to the vertebral bodies that provides cushioning and space between the vertebral bodies and which helps hold them together

Axis, *C1 vertebra,* ring-like vertebra that joins neck to skull

Odontoid process of C2 vertebra, projecting tongue of bone that allows for neck rotation

Luscha joints, connecting joints of cervical vertebrae

Spinal Cord, starts at the base of the brain and stops at the first lumbar vertebra, carries motor and sensory nerves to the extremities and trunk

Spinal Nerve Roots, exit through openings in spine, **foramen,** to supply innervation to muscle, skin, ligaments and joints

Dura, thick protective covering over the brain and spinal cord

Epidural, the location just external to the outer surface of the dura

Spinal fusion, a joining together of a spine segment to another with bone

Dislocation, abnormal position of one vertebra in relationship to the other

Osteotomy, cutting of bone

Stabilization, to rebalance and "shore-up"

Ablation, interventional destruction of a nerve or nerve branch

Implant, a replacement or stabilization part; for example, a disc replacement or a plate and screws

Instrumentation, implants used to hold correction and stabilize the spine, for example pedicle screws coupled with rods

NSAIDs, Non- steroidal anti-inflammatories drugs

CT Scans, Computerized tomography, a type of x-ray that allow three-dimensional (3D) visualization of the spine

MRI, Magnetic Radiographic Imaging, uses high strength electromagnets rather than radiation to image the spine

DEXA, Dual Energy X-ray Absorption scan uses low dose X-ray beams to measure bone density.

EMG, **E**lectromyography, used to detect abnormal nerve and muscle function by sampling the response of various muscles and nerves to signals from the brain.

NCT, **N**erve **C**onduction **T**ests, uses electrical stimulation to evaluate whether or not the nerve is transmitting signals properly and at what speed

SSEP, Somatosensory Evoked Potentials, method of monitoring the sensory function of the spinal cord and nerves to electrical stimulation during surgery

MEP, Motor Evoked Potentials, measurements of the motor function of the spinal cord and nerves to electrical stimulation during surgery

Acknowledgements

We cannot possibly thank everyone who helped and inspired us along the way. Our wives have steadfastly stood beside us. They have been there for us on many family occasions when we were caring for patients. We thank them from the bottom of our hearts. Without them, our careers and our lives outside of work would have been meaningless.

We owe a profound thanks to those who helped educate us: our teachers in grammar school, high school, university, and medical school, and the professors and support staff in our orthopaedic training programs who gave so much of themselves to help us learn and understand our profession.

Special thanks to Madeline White, a junior premedical student at Virginia Polytechnical Institute, Dick's grandniece, for her time and talent expended in producing the meaningful illustrations.

We deeply appreciate our volunteer readers who worked diligently to help make this book more readable, Ed Hearn, Diane Torgerson, Al Wordsworth, John Roper, and Bryan Noah. A very special thanks to Marie Gillis for doing the final edits and proofing.

Any errors you may find are ours, but without our readers there would be many more.

Finally, we are most appreciative of your reading this work. As it is the fourth in a series with more to come, we would like to hear from you about what you like and do not like, so we can try to improve with each book.

Posting a candid review on Amazon would be most appreciated.

Printed in Dunstable, United Kingdom